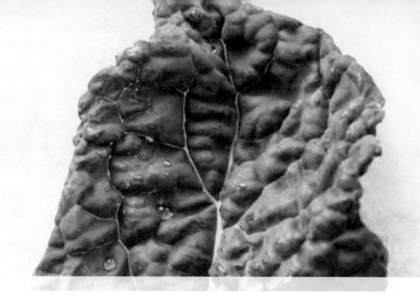

EAT YOUR WAY
TO
Gut-Health

RESTORE GOOD GUT-HEALTH THROUGH THE FOODS YOU EAT DAILY

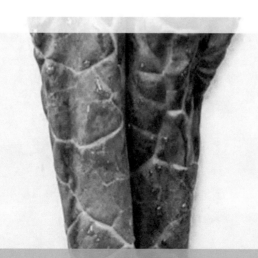

ROSA BUNN

Table of *Contents*

Introduction to the
COOKBOOK

"Regain life-energy through the food you eat daily"
- this sentence has been the inspiration for writing this cookbook.

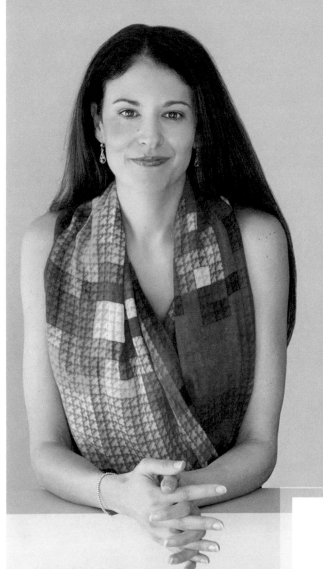

I've dedicated mostly this book to healing and repairing the gut, build good gut flora through foods. Instructions for preparing meals which focus on building your gut flora.

You will find ways to help you learn more about prebiotic foods, probiotic foods and learn the cooking methods of combining foods to assist in growing good gut flora to improve digestion.

By achieving good digestion, you will benefit greatly from the foods you eat, your absorption will be better, your gut lining will have enhanced integrity, overall, this will promote good health, have the potential to assist in slowing disease states, have the potential to aid in the recovery of disease states.

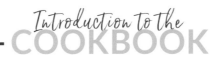

Mindful eating is simply being mindful whilst eating your food.

It is having your full presence to the food you are about to eat, it's actually seeing your food, seeing the colour, noticing the texture, tasting each mouthful, experiencing the texture of the food etc.

It is also the practical nature of switching off from all devices, television, iPads, laptop, smartphones.

The focus becomes on what you are putting in your mouth, in your body.

Unplug and focus into what you are doing with the first step of food shopping, food preparation, understand the type of foods you are choosing & be mindful on this step.

Be mindful on how you are eating, the quantity of food you are eating, your portion size, control your desires, listen to your stomach, your body for signals you've forgotten to hear, look at the actual piece of food, see it for its beauty, study and be curious about your food.

Learn the nutrient values, learn about it's origin, be curious about where it was grown, how it was harvested, notice the texture of the food, bite and chew your food slowly, swallow the food and follow it down to your stomach.

Allow the relationship of the food to be establishment so you can feel nourishment from the food you eat.

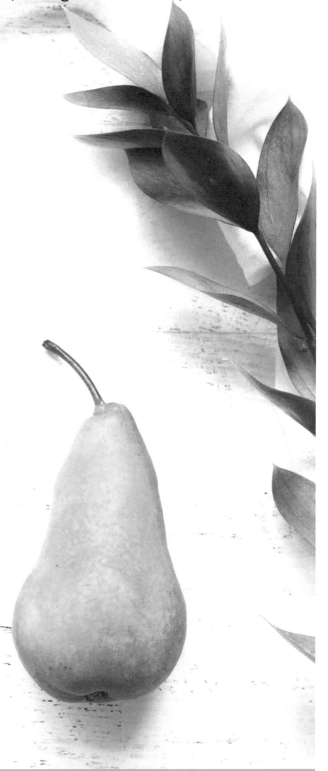

Thanks and acknowledgements-

So many people have been part of my journey to arrive here, to be given the opportunity to present this cookbook to you.

Firstly, my beautiful late Grandma Ida for everything she showed me, the most important key ingredient to cooking & preparing food is love.

The love for preparing food for yourself and for your loved ones. The love you feel in working with the food you are handling.

Thanks to my Mother Gina, for her inspiration of selecting the best ingredients possible, her rapport building skills with farmers, local produce, local fruit shop, local butcher etc, for always selecting the freshest ingredients.

Her passion and her joy from being in the kitchen still inspires me daily. I hear her singing in her kitchen and her proud sense of self coming through as the food is presented.

Thanks to my clients who inspire me weekly to their own commitments for their own personal health. Thank you for your commitment & dedication.

Sending you love and care.

Here's to having good meals, each and every day which build good gut flora!

Rosa xo

A small note on the photographs - the photos are my own mostly. I have enjoyed over the last 4 years collecting my favourites. I hope this inspires you & you are able to select a few favourites to make these part of your weekly food preparation.

About the
AUTHOR

ROSA BUNN, IS A LEADER IN HER FIELD, A QUALIFIED CLINICAL NUTRITIONIST, SPECIALISING IN NUTRITIONAL MEDICINE. SHE RUNS A FUNCTIONAL MEDICINE, INTEGRATIVE MEDICINE CLINIC. HER 15 YEARS OF CLINICAL EXPERIENCE HAS BROUGHT GREAT KNOWLEDGE WHICH SHE SHARES DAILY WITH HER CLIENTS.

ROSA ALSO HOLDS AN ADVANCED HERBAL MEDICINE QUALIFICATION, WORKING HANDS ON WITH BOTANICALS, HER RANGE OF BOTANICA IS DESIGNED TO TREAT CHRONIC DISEASE STATES, PAIN MANAGEMENT, ANXIETY, INFLAMMATION, GUT-REPAIR, BUILD AND MAINTAIN GOOD GUT FLORA, IMMUNE REPAIR.

ROSAS' BACKGROUND OF HER TEACHING QUALIFICATIONS IN PILATES AND ALSO IN YOGA MEANS THAT SHE SPECIALISES IN BODY REPAIR AND REGENERATION THROUGH THE MIND-BODY DISCIPLINES OF PILATES, YOGA, MEDITATION, BREATHE EXERCISES. ROSA HAS SEEN THAT CHRONIC DISEASE STATES DEPLETE THE NATURAL RESERVES OF THE BODY. FUNCTIONAL MEDICINE, INTEGRATIVE MEDICINE, AS A COMPREHENSIVE, COMBINED APPROACH ASSIST IN REBUILDING THESE CRUCIAL RESERVES FOR ACHIEVING A BETTER QUALITY OF LIFE.

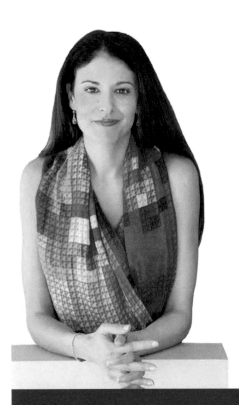

This cookbook is intended to give you a taste of my work and provide you with a glimpse to the mindset behind the recipes, the art of repair and regeneration of the healing mechanics of the body.

It is with great pleasure I present this to you, I hope it provides you with structure and helps you get organised and allows you to start living a better life for yourself. I wish you all the best in your health and wellbeing.

Please connect: rosa@regainenergy.com.au
Instagram @rosabunn
Facebook @regainenergy

PANTRY LIST

What you need to get prepared

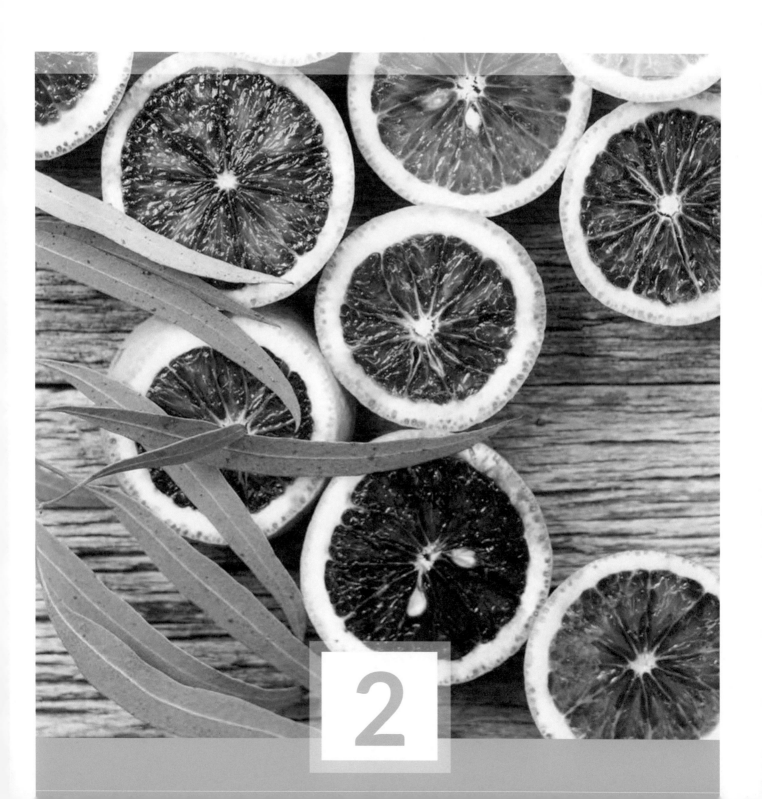

2

What's in the fridge? A new concept of the "cold pantry".

**Fresh wholesome foods. Start thinking about where these come from..
Where's the source of your food coming from?**

Who in your local community are organic farmers, look for fresh organic produce, start with some key essentials such as organic eggs, fresh organic milk, almond milk, key organic green vegetables such as broccoli, green beans, spinach, garden leaf greens, citrus fruits for example lemons, oranges, green apples, herbs, key ingredients.

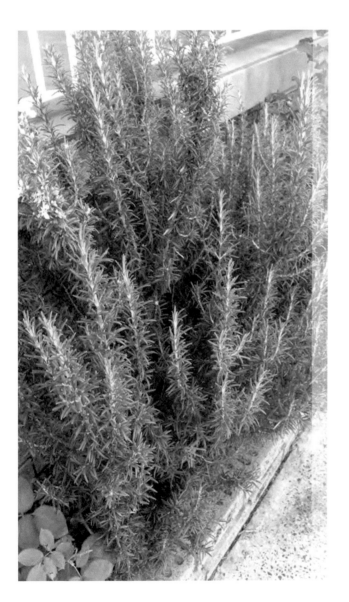

Let's start with planting herbs in pots, you can have these sitting on your kitchen bench, small area on the balcony such as a garden wall.

Great herbs to start with include:

- Basil
- Mint
- Parsley
- Coriander
- Rosemary
- Dill
- Thyme

The mindset of pantry list changes from dried, processed ingredients to a new way forward that includes fresh ingredients that are primarily found in the fridge or garden/ earth.

PANTRY LIST
What you need to get prepared

Pantry Contents

Earth foods such as....

- Potatoes
- Sweet potatoes
- Onions
- Lemons
- Bananas
- Tomatoes
- Pumpkin seeds
- Sunflower seeds
- Almond meal
- Rolled oats
- Quinoa
- Brown rice
- Basmati rice
- Teff
- Kasha toasted buckwheat groats

- Chia seeds
- Acai powder
- Raw cacao
- Organic raw cacao nibs
- Molasses
- Tamarind
- Cloves
- Soy sauce
- Tamari
- Fish sauce
- Chocolate
- Slippery elm
- Organic coconut flakes
- Fish Sauce

- Chocolate
- Slippery elm
- Organic coconut flakes
- Avocados
- Coconut oil
- Cinnamon
- Local raw organic honey
- Pink Himalayan salt
- Organic apple cider vinegar
- Maple syrup
- Rapadura sugar
- Stock/broth
- Spices such as black pepper
- Organic black leaf tea
- Green tea

Make your own teas using fresh ingredients such as ginger tea, turmeric lattes, golden milk, chai tea; healing teas such as basil tea, camomile tea, lemongrass tea & fresh ingredients from your own pantry, fridge and kitchen.

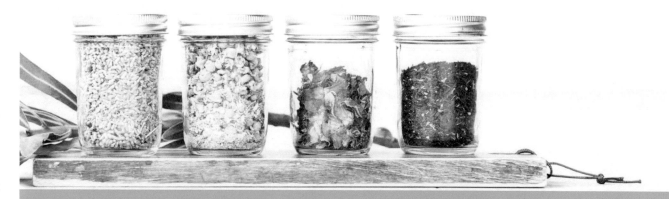

WHAT'S IN THE FRIDGE

"Cold Pantry"

THE FRIDGE SHELVES FROM TOP TO BOTTOM LOOK LIKE THIS...

Top Shelf

Eggs, organic grass fed produce such as butter, milk, goat's cheese and feta (in moderation), prebiotic foods such as kimchi - fermented cabbage and fermented vegetables (detailed in the section of prebiotic foods), white miso paste, cashew hummus, beetroot hummus, tempeh

Second Shelf

Greek yoghurt (full fat), natural coconut yoghurt, seeds for example, linseeds, some oils are olive oil, flaxseed oil & macadamia oil

Third Shelf

Fruit such as oranges, apples, berries, seasonal fruits, pomegranate, pears fresh spices such as ginger & turmeric, aloe vera

Fourth Shelf

Vegetables can be celery, carrot, red and green peppers, lettuce, broccoli, asparagus, snow peas, zucchini - white and green, yellow squash, cucumbers, snow pea sprouts, all sprouts, beetroot

Freezer

Stock/broths, frozen berries, frozen lemons, white miso

Drinks

Water recipes, fresh juices, fresh smoothies, preserve pre-made fresh juice with vitamin C powder to last 2-3 days, coconut water, Kombucha drinks, vinegar drinks, cold kitchen made teas

Treats

Treats can be organic raw cacao nibs, almonds, cashews, brazil nuts, walnuts, seeds, coconut flakes, raw cacao, organic chocolate, organic red wine, homemade chips such as kale, beetroot, sweet potato, potato with skins, hummus, dips/chia sees puddings, organic chocolate mousse (guar gum and inulin fibres which feed good gut flora which can be added to chocolate mousse and other recipes)

HERBS
Essential Key Ingredients

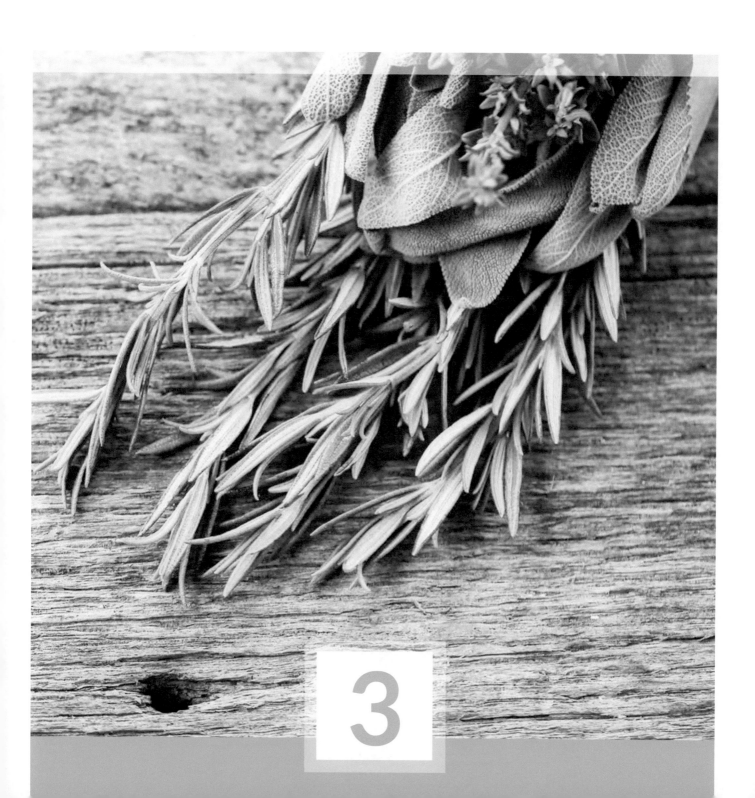

3

HERBS
Essential Key Ingredients

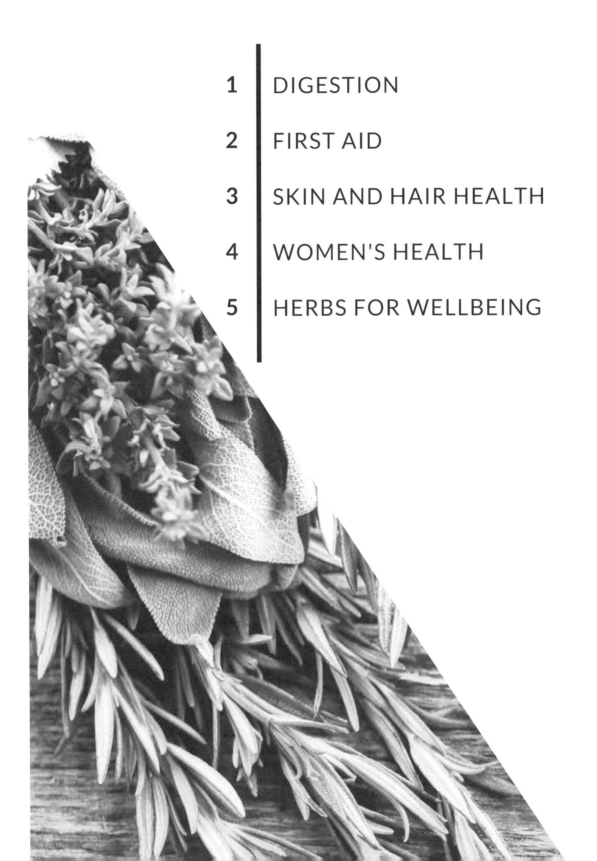

HERBS
Essential Key Ingredients

Digestion

Fennel

Aids with indigestion, wind and constipation

Peppermint

Aids indigestion, flatulence, irritable bowel syndrome

Camomile

Aids digestion, calms stomach

Meadowsweet

Aids gastritis, upset stomachs, avoid in pregnancy or if sensitive to aspirin

Marshmallow

Aids indigestion. alleviate Crohn's disease

First Aid

Marigold — Antiseptic, easy to eat with rice, eggs, salad leaves, fish, chicken

Camomile — Aid digestion, insomnia, soothes stomach aches, easy to eat with apricots, peaches, strawberries, honey, lemon and fish

Echinacea — Immune support, mouthwash, sore throats, make tea with dried leaves

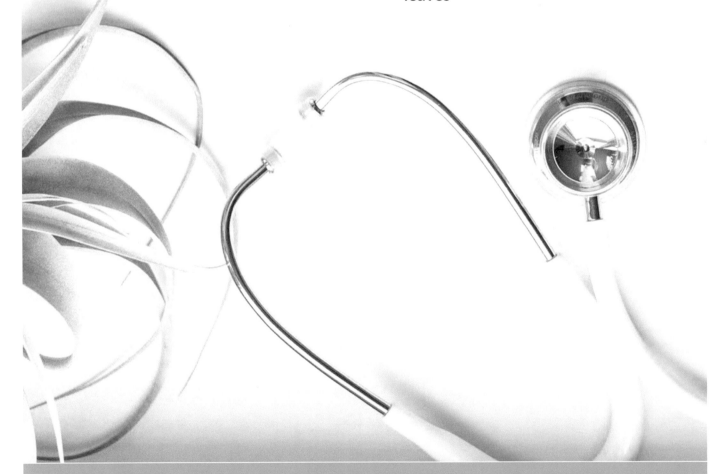

HERBS
Essential Key Ingredients

Skin and Hair Health

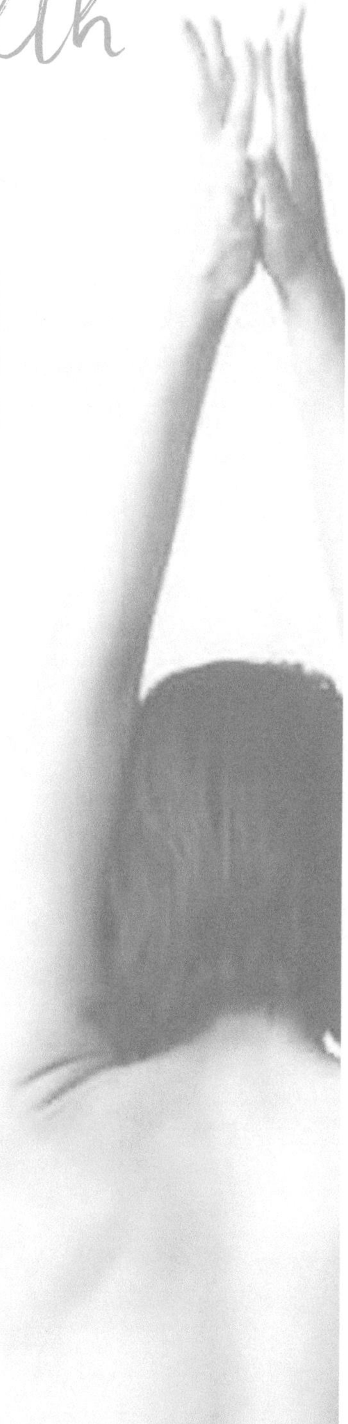

Marigold

Antiseptic for skin pimples, skin infections, easy to eat with salad leaves, rice

Lavender

Good for skin and hair rinse, calming on skin, easy to eat with strawberries, peaches, white fish, goats cheese, thyme, orange and lemon

Nettle

Good for dandruff and hair rinse, useful for eczema, easy to eat with rice, soft cheese, eggs, potatoes, garlic, onions, fish and chicken

Thyme

Antiseptic, easy to eat with leeks, sweet potatoes, squash, carrots, eggs, pasta, orange, lemon, apples

Women's Health

Lady's mantle

Help with eczema, ulcers, sore throats, menstrual pain, breast tenderness

Camomile

Calming, soothing, aids digestion

Rose

Menstrual complaints, calming, anti-inflammatory, rosewater in skin preparations

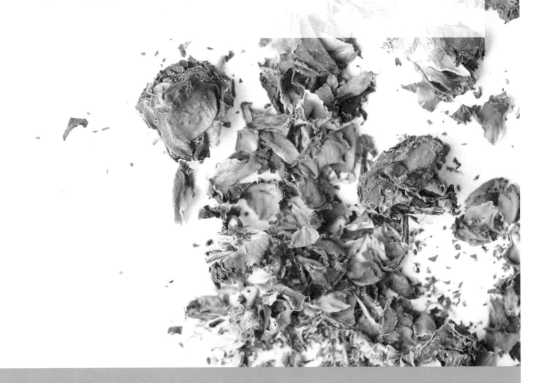

Vervain

Improve digestion, help with stress, anxiety and depression

Herbs for Wellbeing

Rosemary

Good mood, brain clarity, can be taken for tiredness and headaches, eat with peppers, onions, tomatoes, potatoes, cabbage, olives, pears, plums

St.John's Wort

Soothes anxiety, irritability, nervous tension, can be helpful for mild to moderate depression, enhance low mood

Garlic

Boost immune system, aid infections

Sage

Helps digestion, menopausal symptoms, gargle for sore throats, tonsillitis, hair rinse for dandruff. Eat with polenta, green beans, apples, onions, potatoes

Basil

High levels of Vitamin A, antibacterial, anti-inflammatory, high levels of betacarotene, easy to eat with eggs, mint, peaches, strawberries, figs, shellfish

Ginseng

Energising nature of this herb, endurance, rebuilding stamina and strength

Ginko

Aid memory loss, helps reduce varicose veins, aid poor circulation, helps good mood

Camomile

Calming on stomach, calming on digestion, soothing on nervous system

What's for
BREAKFAST?

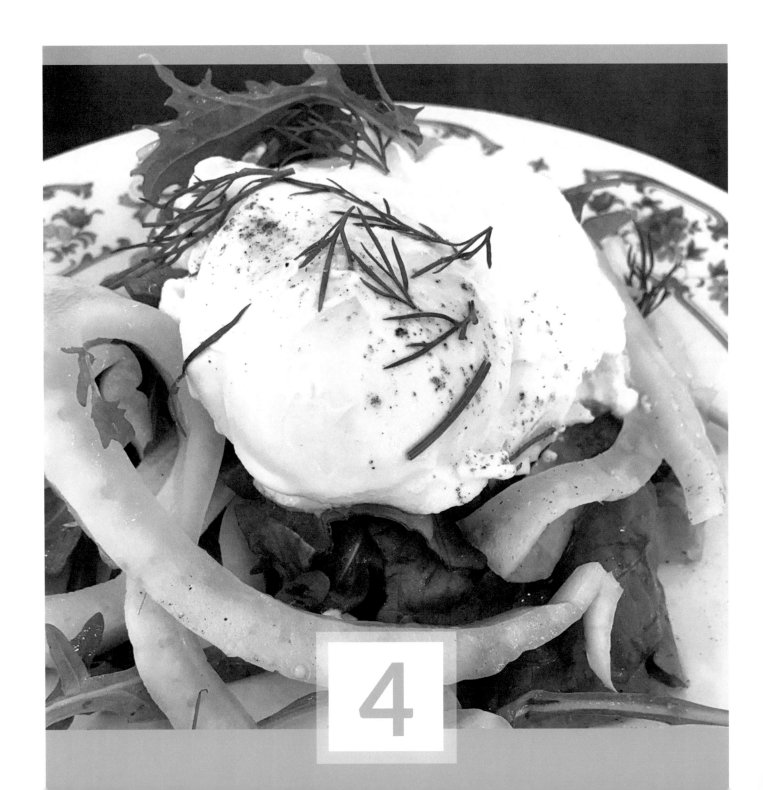

What's for breakfast CAME INTO MY LIFE WHEN MANY OF MY CLIENTS WERE ASKING ME WHAT I WAS HAVING FOR BREAKFAST. ...

I actually started to get really excited about sharing with my clients what i was preparing for breakfast. You see I think breakfast is the most important meal of the day.

It's important because too often we skip it, we miss it, we get on with the day without the food source of what our bodies need and we just grab that quick coffee and just keep going into the day and we may even just grab a small snack for lunch, often I see my clients without any food until the evening meal.

I actually see this a disaster for digestion. The digestion has suffered all day long waiting for food. If the body is waiting for food and it knows through your patterns and your program that you are most likely not to feed it until that night it will save all the energy to allow you to live, this energy is usually stored as fat within the body. It shows up as fat around your stomach, in your legs, your arms, your face etc.

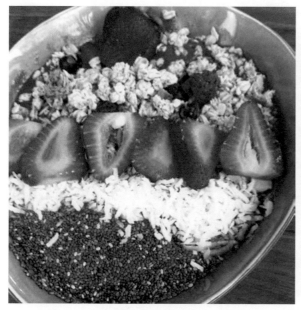

Buddha Bowl

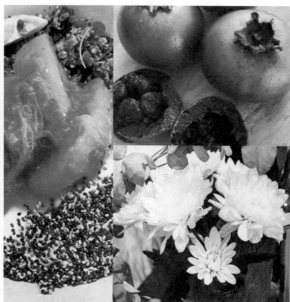

Tropical Fruits

So...What's for breakfast?

Meal suggestions through images to get your creative juices flowing, I want the meals to be simple and easy to prepare.

You select what's in your omelette, what's in your buddha bowl, you chose your ingredients that you love and want to eat more of.

Here's the thing, at first you are so removed from whats actually good for you that you crave all the things which are bad for you like ice-cream, cakes, sweets, soft-drinks.

This isn't about forcing a change for you. It's the stage where you are ready and want to jump in and start making great food for yourself.

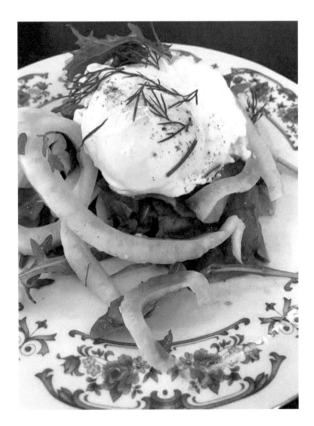

Poached Egg & Fennel Salad

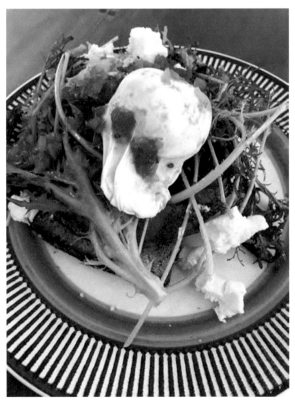

Poached Egg & Salad

Breakfast
RECIPE

Here's an amazing meal with the concept of a
Buddha bowl for breakfast:-

1 STIR-FRY IN COCONUT OIL, CARROTS AND ZUCCHINI, CUT INTO RIBBONS, COOK UNTIL TENDER

2 MAKE THROUGH ABSORPTION METHOD QUINOA ADD 1/2 CUP TO BUDDHA BOWL

3 PREPARE 1/4 OF AVOCADO, MASH AVOCADO

4 BEETROOT HUMOUS, BOUGHT ORGANIC OR MAKE YOUR OWN BY BOILING ORGANIC BEET UNTIL TENDER, BLEND, PUREE BEET WITH A HINT OF GREEK YOGURT OR CASHEW NUT BUTTER

5 MIXED GREEN LEAVES & SPROUTS, CHOOSE WHAT YOU ENJOY

6 COCONUT CLUSTERS, ROLL ORGANIC COCONUT FLAKES WITH COCONUT BUTTER INTO BALLS AND PAN-FRY INTO CLUSTER, YOU CAN ALSO BAKE THESE SEPARATELY

7 TEMPEH, MARINATED TEMPEH, MARINATE TEMPEH OVERNIGHT WITH YOUR FAVOURITE INGREDIENTS, SPICES

8 LEMON, ADD REAL LEMON JUICE AND SHARE THIS OVER YOUR BUDDHA BOWL TO START THE TINGLING OF LIVE ENZYMES TO START YOUR DIGESTION.

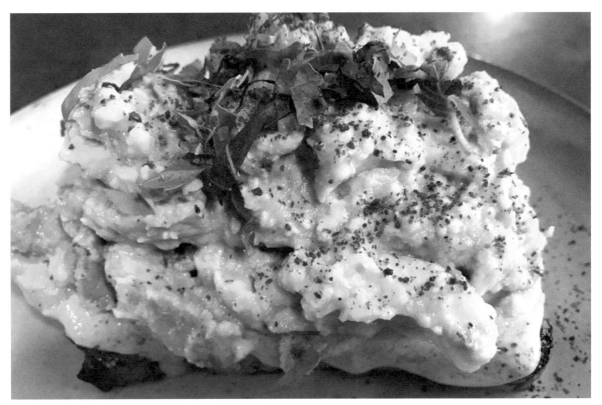

Healthy Omelette

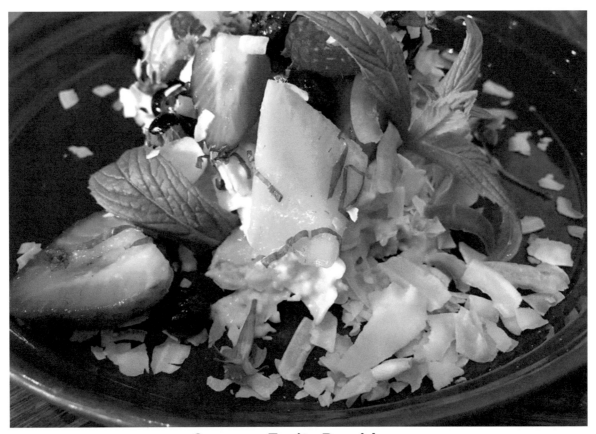

Summer Fruits Porridge

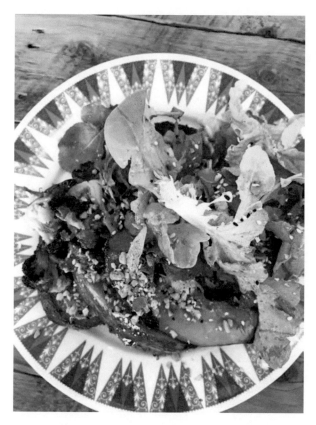

Baked Pumpkin & Salad

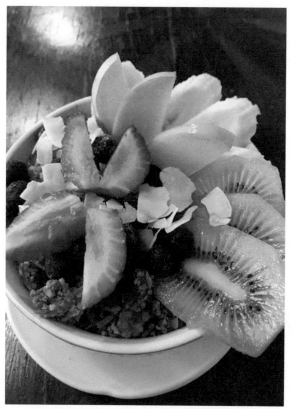

Fruit bowl Seeds & Yogurt

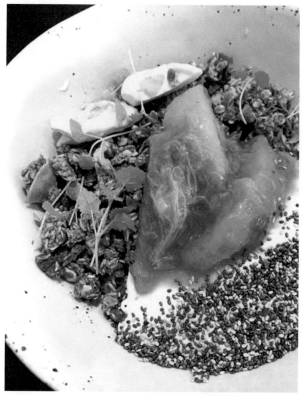

Breakfast Poached Fruits

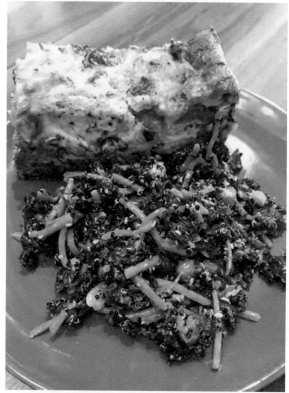

Quiche & Quinoa Salad

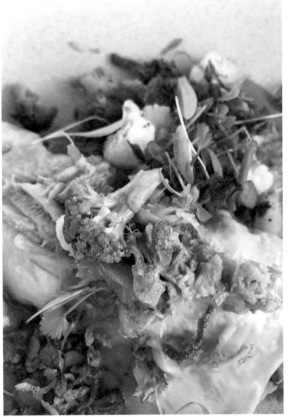

Vegetable Cauliflower Omelette

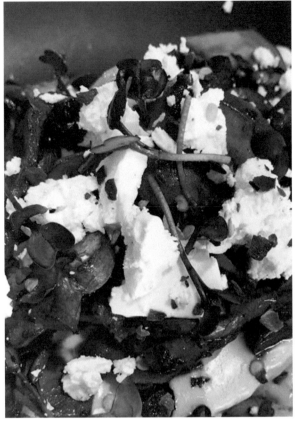

Mushroom Toast

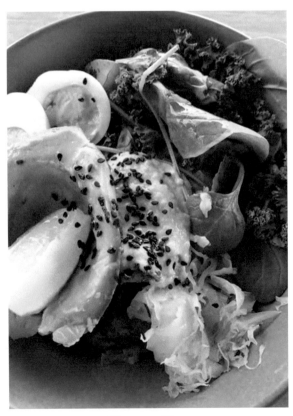

Green Eggs

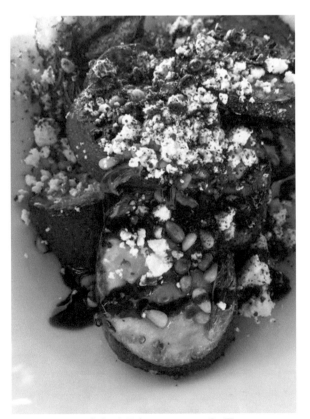

Zucchini Pinenuts & Feta

Sources of
PREBIOTIC
FOODS
& drinks

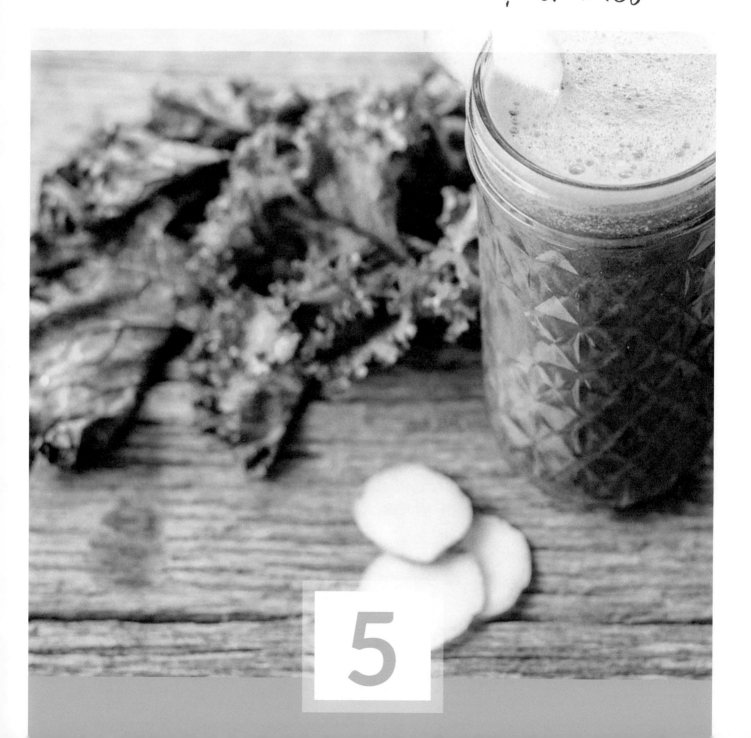

5

Prebiotic Sauces & Drinks

These are foods prepared in the kitchen with fresh ingredients that are food to your gut flora...

For example, kimchi, kombucha, white miso, buttermilk, fermented bean paste, pickling, pickled foods, tempeh, Worcestershire sauce, tabasco sauce, Greek yoghurt, chicken broth, beef-bone broths, stock/broths.

Gut flora, gut microbiota is also referred to as gastrointestinal microbiota. This is a complex community of micro-organisms that live in our digestive tracts.

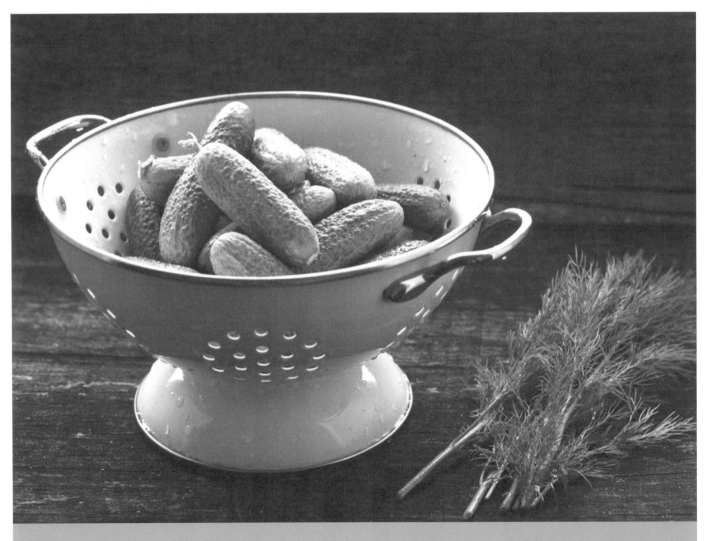

Recipes &
INGREDIENTS

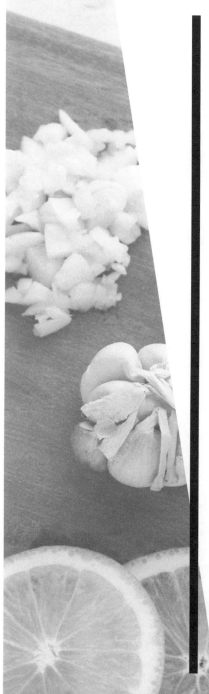

Worcestershire Sauce
KITCHEN MADE (HOMEMADE)

Ingredients
- Malt vinegar
- Molasses
- Sugar
- Salt
- Tamarind extract
- Onions
- Garlic
- Cloves
- Soy sauce
- Tamari
- Fish sauce
- Lemons
- Pickles and peppers
- Add pureed apple, tomato, maple syrup

All quantities to your taste.

Start with a balance of a tablespoon of each ingredient and then adjust this accordingly to your taste.

It's a great way to get creative and start thinking about ingredient blending.

Kimchi
FERMENTED SIDE DISH, WHICH CAN BE ADDED IN ANY MEAL
KITCHEN MADE (HOMEMADE)

Ingredients
- Medium sized cabbage
- 1/4 cup red chilli
- 1 tablespoon minced garlic
- 1 tablespoon ginger
- 3-4 onions
- 2 tablespoons fish sauce
- 1/2 apple
- 1/4 cup sea salt
- Water

Method
Chop cabbage into bit-sized pieces, sit cabbage in bowl of warm salted water for 4 hours.

Make chilli paste and combine with cabbage, add other ingredients & mix through well. Transfer into fermenting jar, cap tightly.

Ferment for 24 hours at room temperature.

Refrigerate for use.

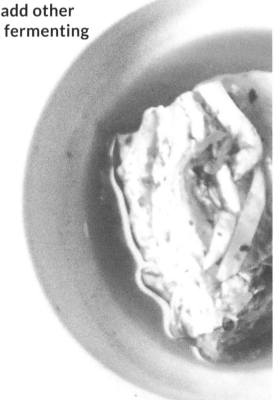

Pickling

PICKLING HAS A 4000 YEAR HISTORY, SO MUCH KNOWLEDGE OF THIS PROCESS OF "PICKLING" IS GOOD FOR GUT FLORA. FERMENTATION PICKLING IS PART OF THE PICTURE FOR GUT HEALTH, BUILDING GOOD GUT FLORA.

Method

Fruits and/or vegetables are placed into a sterile jar along with brine, vinegar or broth. Spices and herbs are added.

The food is then left to ferment until the desired taste is obtained.

In fermentation pickling, the food itself produces the preserve agent involving "lactobacillus" bacteria that produce lactic acid as the preserve agent.

That's why pickles are a source of healthy probiotic microbes.

It's a key step for eating healthy. Achieving good microbiota is the key to achieving good health.

Prebiotic Drinks
RECIPE

Fermented green smoothie with chia seeds

(add 1 teaspoon of fermented yogurt & 1/4 teaspoon of apple cider vinegar, for fermentation)

Soak 5 tablespoons of chia seeds in full glass of water
5 kale leaves or spinach leaves
Chop, 1 banana
Blueberries (optional)
Strawberries (optional)
Lemon
Ginger
Pear or apple
500ml water
Add parsley or herb to you taste
Add honey for sweetness for your taste.

Blend all ingredients and drink this in the morning upon rising, allow this to sit in your gut for at least 20-30mins before eating your breakfast meal.

Prebiotic Drinks
RECIPE

Fermented turmeric, ginger & honey drink

(add pickled turmeric, grated & soaked in brine or malt vinegar)

Grate fresh turmeric, ginger root, add honey to taste, add hot water to these ingredients in teapot.

Steep from 30mins to an hour before drinking.

Add basil leaves to the mixture for extra medicinal benefits of anti-bacterial, anti-viral properties, a great drink which aids in lowering inflammation in the bowel, calming state on digestion tract, soothing qualities.

Good for calming acid reflux, good for settling the stomach.

BUDDHA BOWLS

why these are so valuable to health

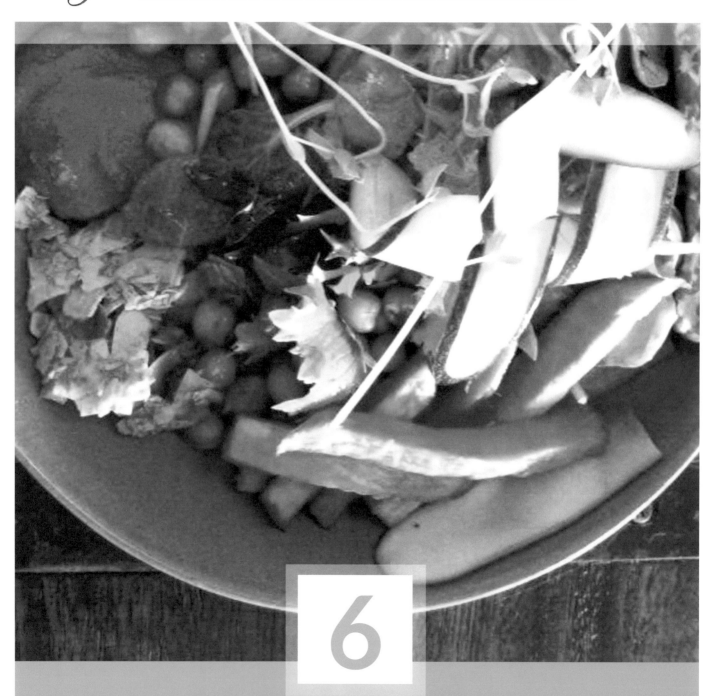

6

BUDDHA BOWLS

& why these and so valuable to health

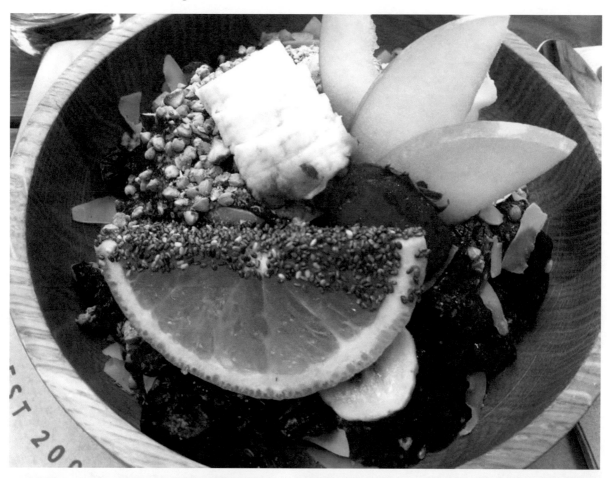

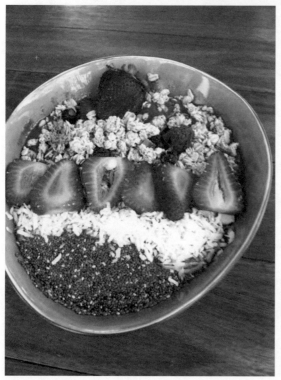

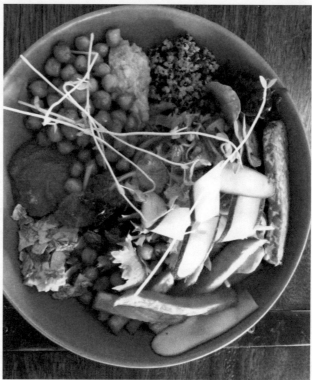

BUDDHA BOWLS
& why these and so valuable to health

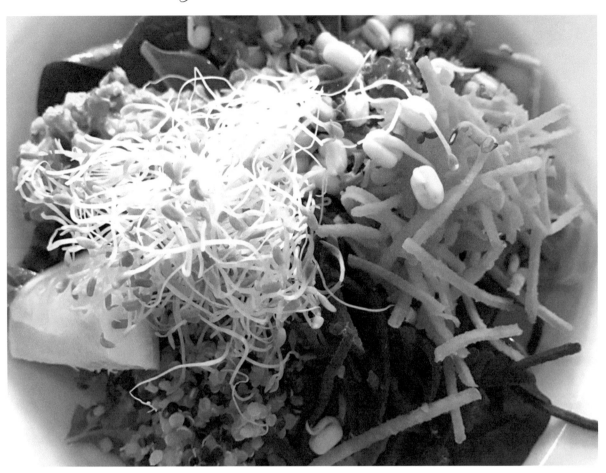

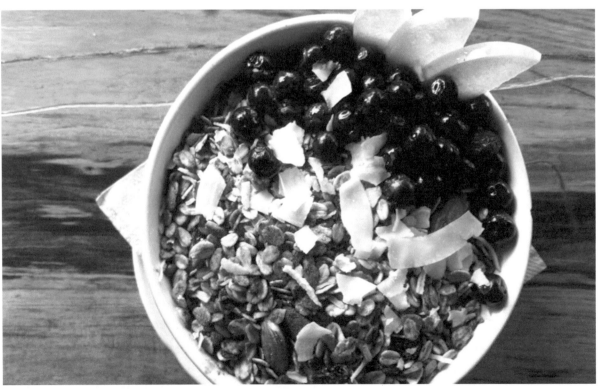

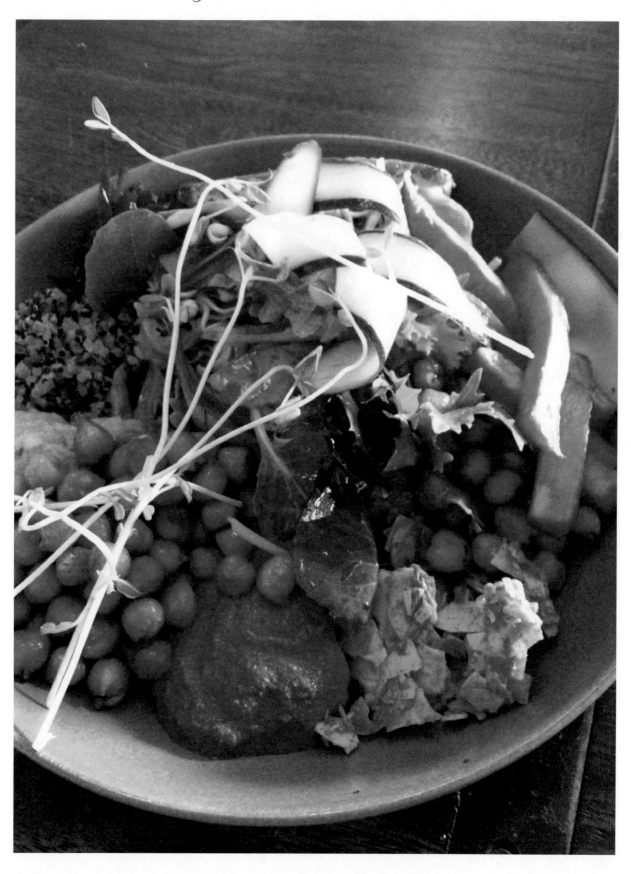

Revive your
FLORA

steps on how to grow good gut flora

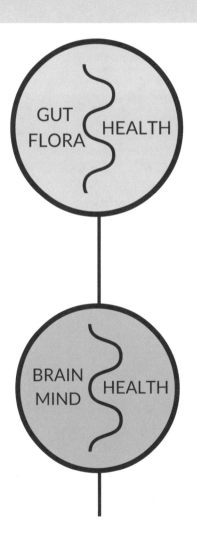

PROBIOTICS
for your gut repair

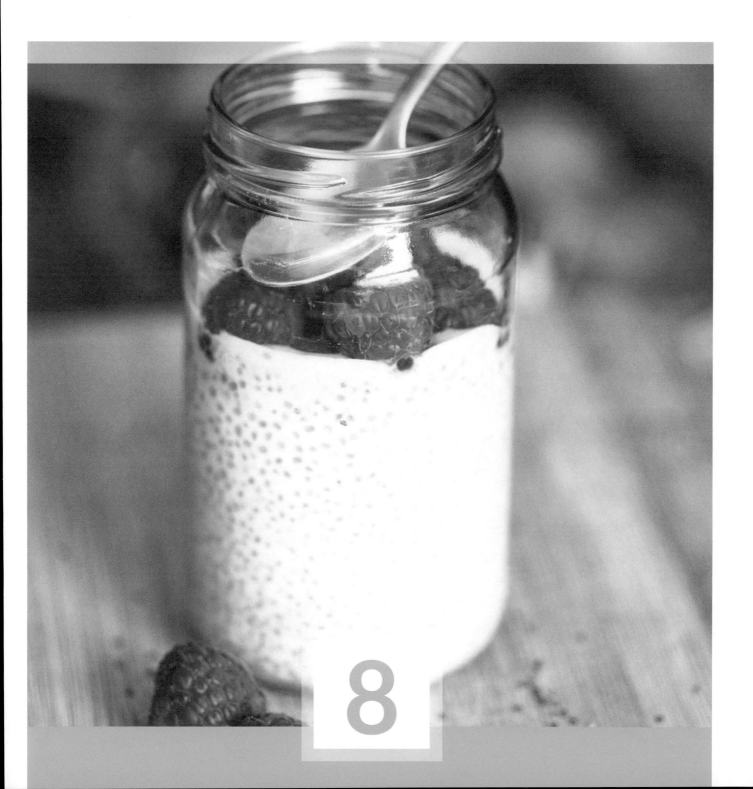

SOUPS
vegetable soups for energy

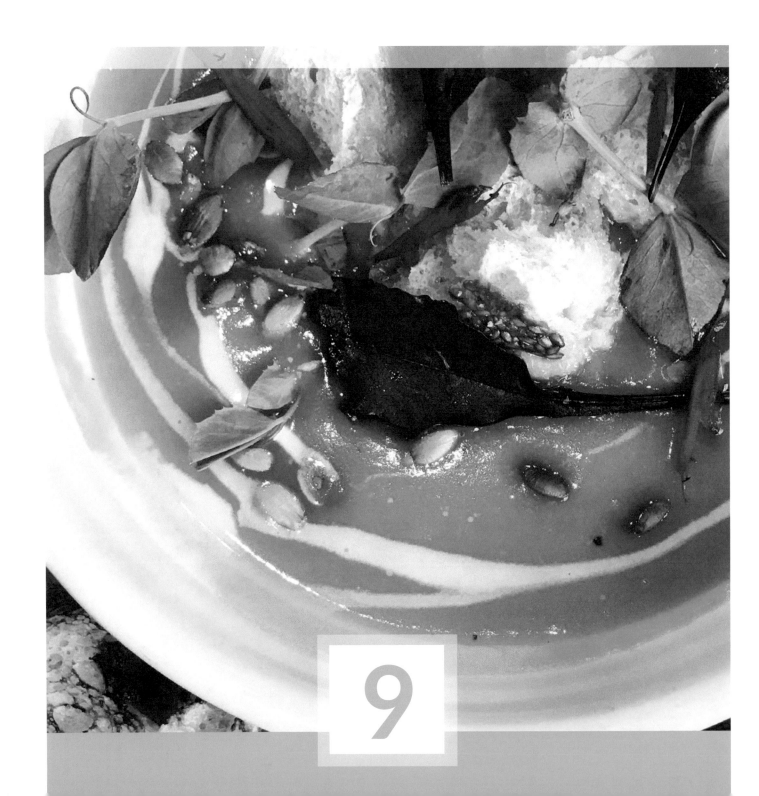

9

Antioxidant Soup PROMOTES GUT HEALING THROUGH SLOW COOKED FOODS BLENDED TOGETHER. EASIER ABSORPTION FOR THE GUT. THIS IS ESPECIALLY IMPORTANT FOR REGENERATION AND REPAIR OF THE BODY

Examples of this include convalescence overcoming the flu, fighting onset of viruses, illnesses, diseases, cancer treatment. Soups have a supportive role in food intake, this can be the case when experiencing illness and presentation of poor or low appetite is experienced.

Soups can be made from a seasonal range of vegetables.
Kale, spinach, onions, potatoes, sweet potato, parsnips, turnips, root vegetables are great as winter seasonal vegetables.

You can also embrace themed soups, such as "green minestrone" soup, onion soup, potato and sweet potato soup, organic chicken soup with buckwheat noodles or rice noodles, meat balls soup. These meals can be easy to prepare and require only a minim amount of cooking time.

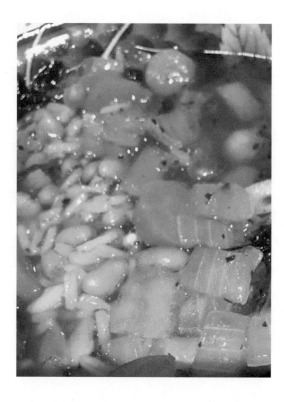 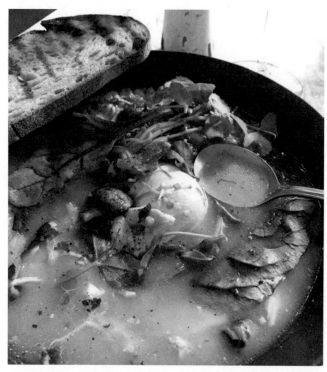

Soup
RECIPE

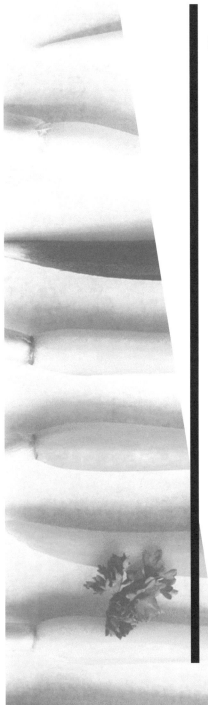

Leek, sweet potato and carrot soup

Ingredients
- 2 litres of water
- Onions
- Garlic
- Carrot
- Leek
- Sweet potato
- Parsley Salt
- Olive oil

Method
Place the cut up mouth size pieces of sweet potato, carrot, leek, onion, garlic, herbs you enjoy like parsley, add another herb you enjoy eating (oregano) in this step here, in 2 litres of water, bring to boil, and simmer for 20-30mins.

Add more herbs, add salt and pepper to taste and olive oil at the end for flavour, just before serving the meal.

Note: add brown rice or quinoa to this vegetable soup if you feel you need a fuller meal.

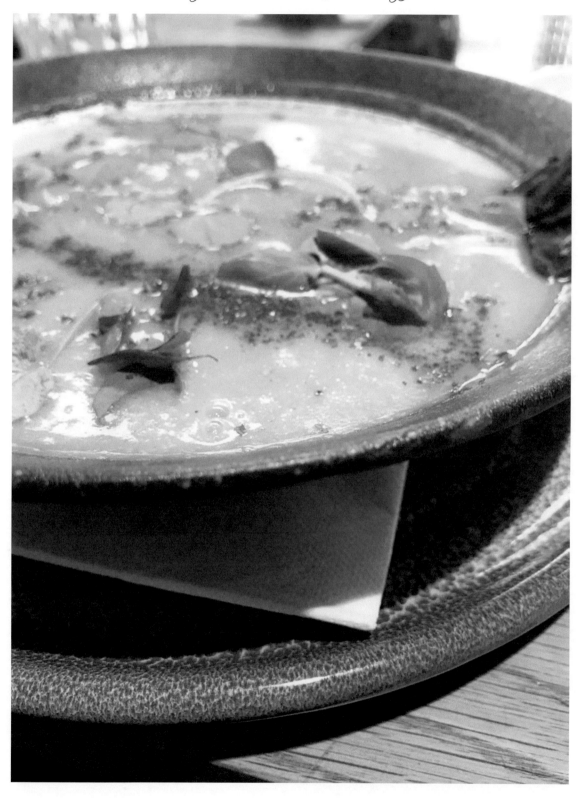

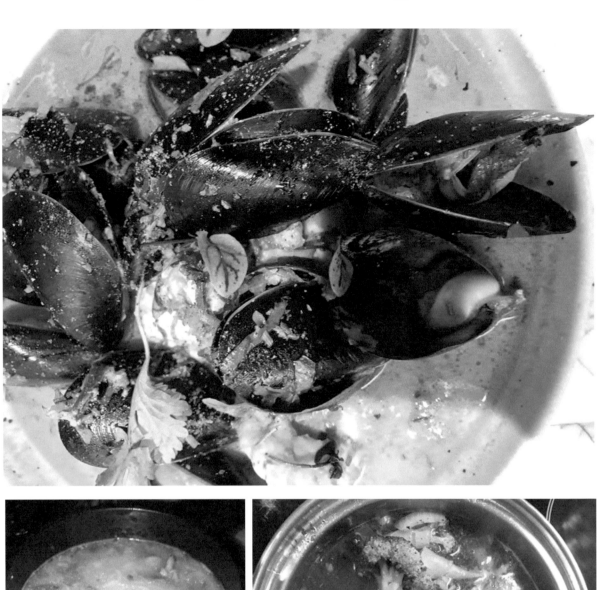

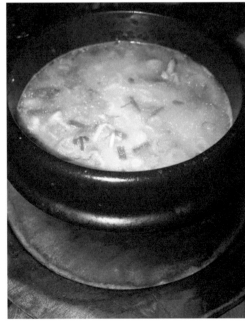

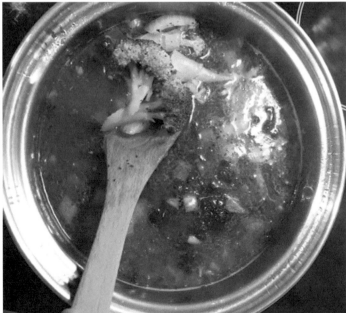

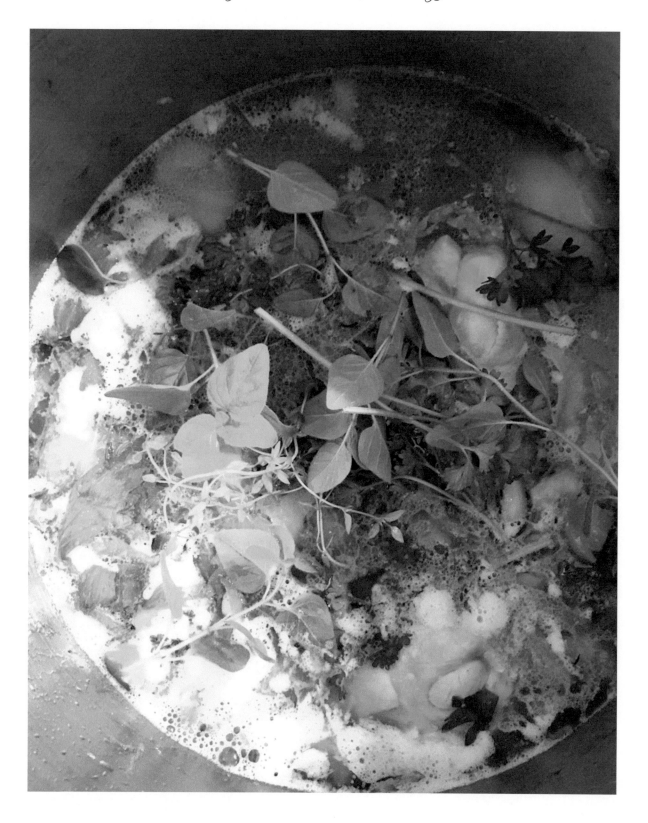

BROTHS
bone broth for healing & repair

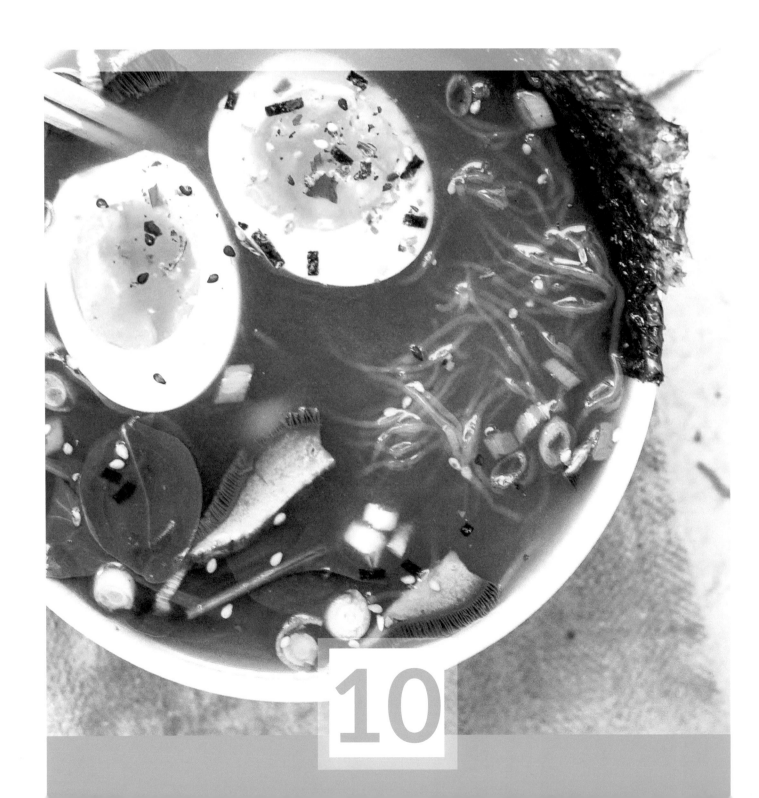

10

Broth
RECIPE

Broth of Chicken
CHICKEN BONE BROTH TO REPAIR GUT INTEGRITY, AID IN REPAIR AND REGENERATION OF THE BODY THROUGH GUT HEALING FOODS

- Brown onion, garlic, carrot, celery, leek, in coconut oil, fry gently until golden in a big heavy pan about 5 litre pan.
- Add organic chicken legs amount 1 per person, brown gently and turn this over so all surfaces are being cooked gently.
- Add water 3 litres or pre-made vegetable stock (this can be the water from boiling vegetables from other meals that you have made in the week), you can also buy fresh packs of stock from health-foods stores and local butchers.
- Bring to the boil, reduce and simmer for an hour until fragrant, add herbs, basil, coriander, thyme, oregano, salt and pepper.
- For an addition to this you can add greens such as English spinach, kale, more herbs, chilli, broccoli, squash etc to make this a variation of the base stock meal of broth of chicken.
- This can be the Mother stock & you can then bring variety to your meals. It is noted that it's the broth of the bone that makes this healing on gut lining and becomes key in gut integrity.
- This soup recipe aids gut integrity and brings repair at the level of essential amino acids.

live enzymes
LIVE FOOD
eating for vitality

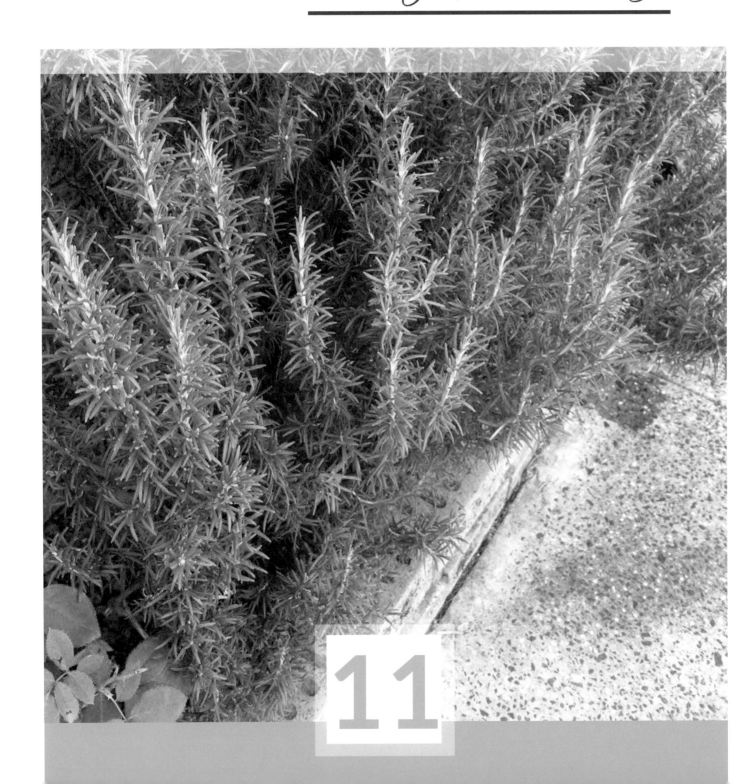

11

Live enzymes
LIVE FOOD
Eating for vitality

Live enzymes, what are they?

These are the live interactions, the active enzymes within the food to help digest 40-60% of that particular food.

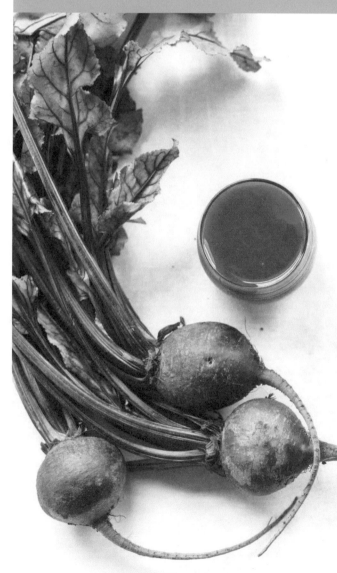

We know that cooking food destroys enzymes, cooked & processed foods are enzymatically dead which means there are no live enzymes within that food to help with digestion.

The signals for digestion, the signals for receiving the food going into your body to start fuelling and nourishing your body are key for digestion.

Without a good digestion system we fall prey to ill health, diseases, malabsorption, lethargy, fatigue, depression, low energy states, chronic illnesses.

Learning and understanding meal prep, learning and understanding live enzymes from the food you eat is a great step forward to achieving good health and creating a fit body which is nourished from a pure foundation.

The food we eat and the food we receive is the first step.

Eating food with live enzymes is a subject which brings me great joy and passion to educate and write about, it's a subject which needs more understanding, education & awareness.

Live enzymes are seen when you first cut through a carrot, the bleed from the carrot on the chopping board is an example of live enzymes from the food you eat.

Without seeing these live enzymes you really aren't eating food which is alive, it's either a processed food or a food that's been reheated or overcooked, basically it's dead food.

The body needs live enzymes to feel the vitality and stay in the vitality state where nutrients are alive and are readily absorbed by the body.

This chapter is to encourage you to eat alive foods, food which are alive, have loads of nutrients coming into your diet to fuel your body.

Your fridge will be your "cold pantry", this is where most of your food will be stored.

This is a new concept for many people to actually see and understand.

We are living further away from the source of our food supply and we are being confused by many marketing fads on what foods we should be eating.

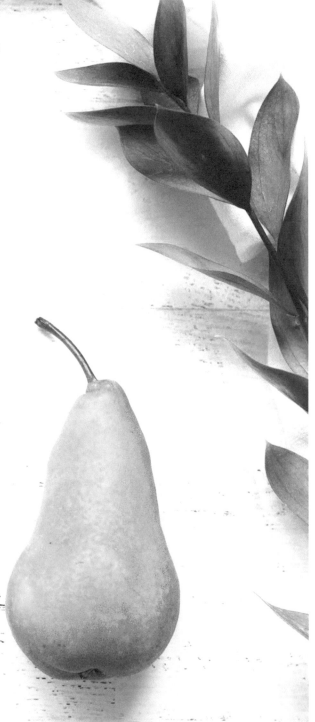

LIVE FOOD

Cutting back, stripping back to the essence of what your body's requirements are is a good approach to changing your diet, your habits and start creating new patterns in the way you handle foods and prepare your foods.

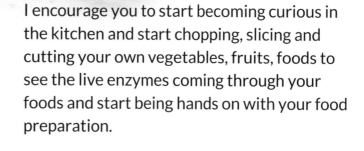

I encourage you to start becoming curious in the kitchen and start chopping, slicing and cutting your own vegetables, fruits, foods to see the live enzymes coming through your foods and start being hands on with your food preparation.

Good gut health starts in your kitchen, your kitchen is your space for looking after yourself, looking after your body, your health and your wellbeing.

It's taking ownership and becoming responsible for the choices you make daily.

Live enzymes, seeing the interaction of the different foods you combine and put together to create the meal for yourself.

The combination of all macronutrients, receiving all the required micronutrients in your diet daily is work, it requires thought, it requires preparation, it requires your commitment to be organised in your week.

COMMUNITY
and collaboration
a network of people to support your health

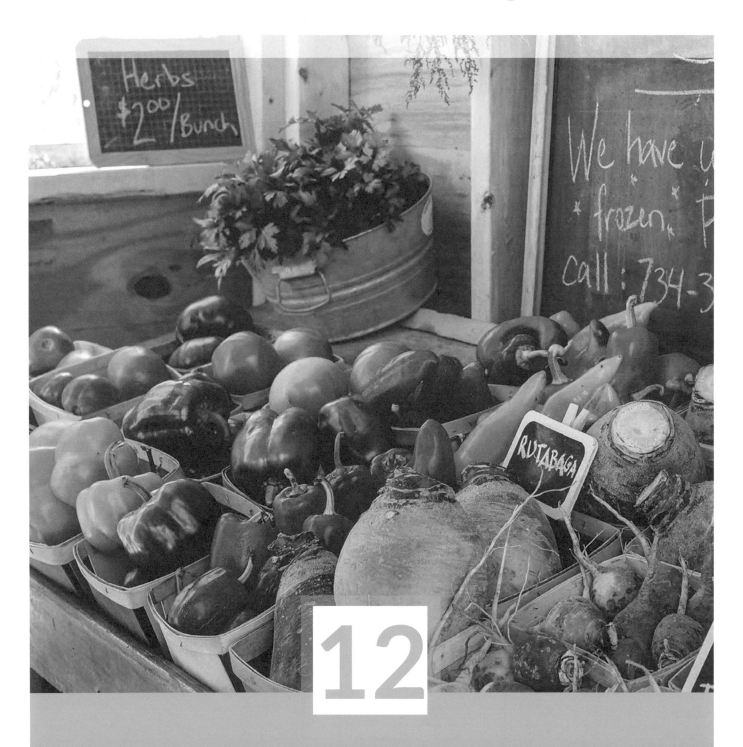

12

COMMUNITY
and collaboration

This section is about community
- the network of individuals which support you to ultimately support and take care of yourself.

The local fruit shop, the local butcher, the local health-food store, the local nutritionist, the local herbalist, the local organics supplier, the local community gardens, farmer's markets, local organic eggs, local honey, just to name a few key areas of food supply.

This network of individuals come together to create a table of ingredients which is shared to make a whole complete meal. The collaboration is required to come together in this setting.

By becoming aware of where your food source is being produced, this gives you greater appreciation of how things are grown, how much time it takes for food to grow. This level of appreciation is required for achieving good sustaining health, it's required for weight loss, it's required to maintain health and wellbeing, allowing you to return to the source of the food.

Some local cafes are producing incredible meals with the theme of whole-foods, they have embraced leadership in the way they prepare your food and allow for food to come together. The concept of Buddha bowls is a great place to start as it demonstrates how a little bit of everything is required to make a meal which is nutrient dense.

There are also online organics which home deliver boxes of vegetables to your door, this is a very convenient way of receiving your food for the week. It's also a very exciting way, an exciting approach.

Balboa Press books may be ordered through booksellers or by contacting:

Balboa Press
A Division of Hay House
1663 Liberty Drive
Bloomington, IN 47403
www.balboapress.com.au
1 (877) 407-4847

Because of the dynamic nature of the Internet, any web addresses or links contained in this book may have changed since publication and may no longer be valid. The views expressed in this work are solely those of the author and do not necessarily reflect the views of the publisher, and the publisher hereby disclaims any responsibility for them.

Any people depicted in stock imagery provided by Getty Images are models, and such images are being used for illustrative purposes only.
Certain stock imagery © Getty Images.

ISBN: 978-1-5043-1818-1 (sc)
ISBN: 978-1-5043-1819-8 (e)

Print information available on the last page.

Balboa Press rev. date: 06/06/2019

BALBOA.
PRESS
A DIVISION OF HAY HOUSE

Printed in the United States
By Bookmasters